Thirty Things About Cancer

A guide to getting through

Dr Mike Goldsmith

**Grammaticus
Books**

This edition first published in Great Britain in 2015 by Grammaticus
Books

ISBN-13: 978-1508549918
ISBN-10: 1508549915

Contents

Introduction

I'm just waiting for the results of my first three-monthly cancer check. A year ago, I was probably waiting for an MRI Scan. Or a CT scan. Or an appointment. Cancer, eh? It sounds dramatic and it can be, but a lot of what it means in reality is waiting for things. It's just one of cancer's many inescapable aspects; but, like the rest of them, it need not be a source of worry or gloom. At least, that is what I've concluded, over more than a year of treatments. There are many things you can do, and many facts you should know, to improve your state of mind and your prospects too. This book introduces thirty of them, and reading them should make you feel at least a bit better. (And *be* a bit better too. Many studies have shown that patients who are better informed and have positive attitudes are more likely to survive cancer).

Who am I?
The only relevant thing I'm an expert on is my own experiences over the two years since I went to my GP with the first symptoms of what turned out to be bowel cancer. I'm not a medical doctor, and the information I've collected has been only through books, the internet, and conversations with health workers and fellow patients. Many, many conversations. Of the roughly four hours average per week I've spent in hospital since I was diagnosed, about two were spent chatting. The thirty things in this book are the result. If I'd known them two years ago, I would have found them very helpful indeed. I hope you do, too.

Who is this book for?
It's for anyone and everyone with cancer. It may be of interest to their families and friends too, and perhaps even to a few health

workers as well (by the way, I use "health workers" to cover all the staff of hospitals, charities, clinics and surgeries with whom you may come into contact).

If you have any comments on this book, or any suggestions as to what to include in the next edition, please do email me at

30thingsabout@gmail.com

There is also a website to accompany this book

http://30thingsabout.weebly.com/

ONE It's a new world

My grandmother died of cancer nearly a century ago - probably. All my dad remembered was that one day she was there at home as usual and the next she was gone, to some distant hospital, with a mysterious disease which no one wanted to discuss. His sisters stepped into her role, my grandfather rarely spoke of her and my father never saw her again. In those days, the very word "cancer" was avoided, and being diagnosed with it was a death sentence, pretty much. On the other hand, it was a relatively rare disease ; the eighth commonest cause of death, compared to the second commonest today (see Facts and stats, page 65). A few decades later, in the 1960s, while so much of the world had changed, the perception of cancer had barely altered. Yet medicine had been revolutionised by new drugs and better care regimes, and cancer survival rates had greatly improved as a result. Nevertheless, because regular tests and checkups were largely unknown and the symptoms of cancer were not well publicised, many people still did not receive cancer treatment early enough to be saved. Also, though surgical techniques were very effective and radiation therapy was increasingly common, recurrence of cancer was a major problem - so, even after cancer had been treated, you still felt you were on a waiting list for death. And the actual treatment could be nightmarish: approaches to surgery were very different then, and emphasised the perceived need for the patient to be denied food or drink for hours, even days, before and after surgery, and to be kept in bed for days afterwards. Now, nurses wave sandwiches and tea at you as soon as you come round and it's a rare patient who is not urged to get up the next day. Another major difference was that until the end of the 20th century, the control of pain was haphazard and unreliable, and a great deal of suffering resulted.

The world of the 1960s still persists – but only in people's heads. Many still hate to use the word "cancer", disregard symptoms, and even ignore doctors, such is the sense of doom associated with the disease. This is little short of a tragedy. In the UK today, the majority of those diagnosed with cancer will survive it. The management of pain is so good that the whole experience can involve none at all. The nature and causes of cancer are now quite well understood and the post-operative treatment is radically different – and far less unpleasant - than it was decades ago. So cancer is by no mean the certain killer it once was, so long as warning signs (see page 56) are not ignored, known cancer-causers like cigarettes (see Causes of cancer, page 57) are avoided, checkups are made, and visits to the GP for further tests are prompt.

The world of cancer has changed in another way too. Today, one in two of us will get it and almost everyone knows someone who has had it. Just a few decades ago, the figure was about 1 in 3. The main reason is that we are living longer, and cancer becomes more likely the older you get. But, though cancer is more likely to knock at your door today than ever before, it is far less likely to become a permanent resident.

When someone is diagnosed with a long term illness, like Alzheimer's, Multiple Sclerosis or Parkinson's, they are usually reminded that in a few years there might be a breakthrough in treatment. Though this is true, such breakthroughs are quite rare – except in the case of cancer. If the last century and especially the last couple of decades are any guide to the future, many breakthroughs will be made. One of many examples is in the treatment of testicular cancer, the commonest type of cancer in young men. Until 1979, survival rates were below 70%, but that year a new drug based on platinum began to be used, and survival rates rocketed. Today, 96% of men who get testicular cancer make a full recovery.

In the 2010s, American scientists tried out a new drug called nivolumab on people with lung cancer (currently the cancer which kills the most people in the UK - about 35,000 annually). The patients involved had advanced forms of the disease, all with life expectances of just a few weeks. Two years later, one-quarter of them were still alive. In one case, the cancer had spread to the patient's liver, brain, bones and adrenal glands when the experimental treatment began. Two years later, there was no trace of cancer anywhere in his body. Trials of this same drug are currently underway in the UK (see the link on page 49 for further information on trials).

Recently, a new family of cancer drugs has been developed, far more targeted than standard chemotherapy drugs are. This means that side effects are often much milder, so, in cases where the cancer can only be controlled rather than removed, drug treatments can continue for many years. Some of these drugs can be taken in pill form at home, and this, combined with the lack of side effects, means that life with cancer could increasingly become like life with high blood pressure, diabetes or HIV: fairly normal, long, and ending in death with cancer rather than death by cancer.

In addition to such promising developments, steady improvement will most likely continue: good chances of cancer survival depend mainly on early and accurate diagnosis, precise surgery, accurate and well-calculated radiotherapy, carefully researched and administered chemotherapy and regular routine follow-ups. All are constantly reviewed and updated, and the effects can be amazing. Someone diagnosed with bowel cancer today, for example, is 17 times more likely to survive than someone diagnosed in 1970. Another example: in 1970, only 25% of men diagnosed with prostate cancer would be alive 10 years later. Now, the figure is 84%. Meanwhile, dealing with side effects has greatly improved – treatment of pain, nausea, hair loss and skin problems are streets ahead of where they were just a decade ago. Many new treatment drugs are being developed, and a great many trials are being carried out. For instance, as I'm writing this there are 127 different trials into breast cancer, of which 82 are looking for people to sign up.

One consequence of all this is that, if you come across some statistic or other about your chances of survival, it is almost certainly pessimistic. "Survival" in cancer terms usually refers to being alive in ten years. Since one can never be certain that cancer will not recur, it's not really possible to say that one has been cured, but the chances of recurrence after five years are small, and after 10 years, recurrence of many cancers is very rare. Of course, the data used to calculate chances of surviving 10 years must necessarily include people diagnosed a decades ago, who did not have the benefits of the progress that has been made since, which can make a significant difference. For instance, in 1971/72, people with leukaemia only had a 6.9% chance of surviving for 10 years. By 2010/11, this had risen to 46.1%, roughly a 10% improvement per decade.

Yet another factor to bear in mind is that those statistics include people who were diagnosed with cancer but opted not to be treated for it, or who abandoned treatment. Though no statistics are available on this, judging by the healthcare people I asked a surprising number of people fall into this category. What is less surprising is that almost all of them died. The published overall survival percentages are therefore lowered.

For the reasons given above, your chances are probably rather better - in some cases, very much better - that whatever statistics you may read.

TWO Look after the people you tell

It's a fair bet that the reactions of the people you tell about cancer will be mixed. Whatever the prognosis, some people (especially older ones), may feel certain you will very shortly be dead and that you are softening the blow by not saying so outright. You may find that whatever else you say after using the word "cancer" will be dismissed by them as "being brave." Some will say, "Oh, I had that." Others will cry. Others will take nothing in once the dread word has been spoken. Some will say "I don't know what to say." Many will offer to help.

The way you deal with these initial reactions is the first stage in looking after the people you tell, and, like so many cancer-related things, it's best to plan your approach in advance - including the medium you will use to let people know. You might decide to email, Skype, text, tweet, update your FaceBook page, do something arty on Instagram, or some other such webby thing. You may even meet them face to face, like people did in the 20th century. Select which you like, but think it through first: if you do meet face to face, it's likely to be a long meeting. If you don't, then tears or other strong reactions will be harder to deal with. Text-based systems allow you to choose your words carefully, but you might be disappointed at the slow response (after all, we're not all permanently always online, are we? Well, I'm not, anyway). On the other hand, a text-based message is likely to lead to a phone-based response; one not at a time of your choosing. Using social media to broadcast your state far and wide should be approached with particular caution. Do you really want everyone you know to know, all at once? Are you even sure who all your FaceBook friends are? Are you prepared to spend the rest of the day answering the phone and hammering responses into your keyboard? Prepare also to have your inbox and FaceBook page suddenly populated by adverts about surviving cancer - or even asking you who will pay for your funeral expenses if you don't (while making a lame attempt to soften the blow by having some celebrity you vaguely remember from a 70's cop show offering you a beautiful carriage clock if you sign up).

However you do it, the relationship between you and those you tell will change, all at once, maybe forever. It could well bring you closer. It may possibly disappoint you (though that's not what I experienced). You might be given advice - which, often being based on decades-old experiences, could be poor.

All the above is no doubt pretty obvious, but what may not be is that you will need to support many of these people. Many of them will want to see you, all of them will want you to keep them informed and quite a lot will need comfort and reassurance. And there will be all sorts of things they will want to know - including things you don't. Although they may not ask you directly, the primary question they will all want answered will be: is it terminal? If you are sure it's not, then this is an easy one to tackle. If you are sure it is, it's probably best to say so, up front, in the first conversation.

Be prepared also to have to repeat many times (within the same conversation, or over many) the facts of your case. You will be familiar with them, and will soon be able to chat like a professional happily about how and why your neutrophil level is hovering around 1.5, but they will not. And to begin with, they will be thinking more about you than the words you say.

One other thing to decide before you tell someone is whether you do or do not wish them to keep the news to themselves.

Bear in mind that, after a while, quite a few people will not *want* to talk about your cancer all the time. You may find your changed bowel habits fascinating, or the lists of possible side effects associated with Oxalyplatin an endless source of interest, but it is just possible that your friends may not. So, remember that the normal rules of polite conversation are not suspended just because you are ill. So, ask your friends how they are, too.

THREE On worrying

The person has yet to be born who, having been diagnosed with cancer, doesn't worry. It is a situation of uncertainty, danger and shock, to which worry is a natural human reaction. But that does not mean to say that the whole of your treatment and your life to come need be full of worry. It's useful to distinguish between natural worry, which can be helpful in prompting the worrier to get things done (sometimes referred to in text books as "concern"), and pointless, self-defeating worry – worry of a kind that prevents the enjoyment of life or which paralyses the mind so that no action is taken.

It is rational to worry about the diagnosis of any serious illness. If such news did not bother people, they would probably not bother much about getting treated for it either, so concern is a very useful reaction. But if you find yourself worrying all or most of the time, if your worrying makes you feel ill, or if you are worrying when actually the news is good, then your worrying is probably excessive.

There are two simple solutions to excessive worrying, which almost always work – though that does not mean they are easy to apply. One solution is psychological and one is chemical, and which works for you depends both on your history and your brain chemistry. If you have a history of excessive worrying, going back before you suspected you might have cancer, then brain chemistry may be the cause. In this case, the solution is to tell your GP, who will probably prescribe you a low-dose course of medication (usually taken once a day, in pill form). If you do try this approach, it is important to stick with it; for one thing it takes several days for the medicine to start changing the brain chemistry, for another, many people find the initial low dose the doctor will prescribe is not enough, and for a third, some drugs work better for some people than others.

If you don't have a history of worrying then the problem is much more likely to be a psychological one. Broadly speaking, excessive worries of this kind are characterised by a reluctance to face a troubling fact or experience, procrastination about making a decision and delay in taking action.

One natural, but usually ineffective, response to a worry is to try not to think about it. But, like anything brushed under a carpet, undercover worries are liable to trip you up – especially in the dark.

Waking with a feeling of general unhappiness, broken sleep or bad dreams are likely consequences.

Sometimes it's hard to pin down exactly what the worry is, but it is important to define it as accurately as possible. Talking it over with a friend is often a help.

Sometimes, simply defining the worry is enough to defuse it, and even if not it is essential for the next step, which is to take a decision. For this stage, be logical, ignore your heart and use your head: that's what it's there for. Again, discussion with others can help a great deal.

And the third stage is : get on with it (or, as a famous sports brand puts it: "Just do it!"). Carry out your decision. Where cancer is concerned, time is very often key, so getting on with things (like going to your GP) could well help your physical health as well as your mental one.

There are other ways of reducing worrying, like frequently repeating to yourself (aloud, if that helps) why the worrying is illogical and/or unhelpful, or setting aside a particular time each day or each week and, when worry strikes, shelving it until that time. The most effective way of dealing with really persistent worrying is a technique called NLP (Neuro-Linguistic Programming). There are books about dealing with worry in the Further Reading Section on page 47.

FOUR Fellow travellers

One thing that makes the treatment of cancer different to that of most other illnesses is that the process takes a long time, and so there will probably be other patients whom you will meet regularly. Unless you feel strongly that you want to soldier on alone, it is well worth talking to them. For one thing, those who have been there longer than you are likely to be mines of useful information, from the quietest time to go for a blood test, to the side effects of treatments, to good books, groups or websites. Secondly, many of the treatments involve a lot of sitting around, and having someone to chat to may make the time go a lot more quickly. Thirdly, these are the people who really do understand what you're going through. There aren't many rules for making friends, but starting by asking a question, taking an interest in the answer and following it up with another question is always a good plan. You can almost always tell at once from the other person's reaction whether they want to talk or not. If not, don't pester them – they may well strike up a conversation with you at some other time. There is just one other "don't": don't assume anything, such as whether they have terminal cancer or not, whether they are religious, gay, depressed or anything else.

FIVE Do your homework

From the moment of your diagnosis, you will be provided with a great deal of information, both verbal and written. And when I say provided, I mean swamped. Overwhelmed, overcome, overburdened. Booklets packed with unnervingly realistic cross sections. Pamphlets full of cancer patients beaming excitedly at the camera, or relaxing happily with their oncologist, as if shortly to wed. Photocopies of articles about everything. Lists and forms, pictures and leaflets, charts and tables. All this will be accompanied by a great many explanations of varying degrees of understandability and comfort. A natural response is to nod sagely , and carefully and tidily put it all in your bag (always have a bag, by the way (that could almost have been a full entry, but it would have been rather a short one)). The huge bundle may well then be put neatly in a box file, on a shelf or stuffed in a drawer of random gubbins, (I'm not saying that's *my* way of filing, you understand), there to remain secure and untouched till you move house. Which is, let's face it, not very useful. Instead, steady your nerves, make some tea and read the stuff. And if you don't understand something, ask. Get yourself in a position where you know what to expect and when to expect it; it really will help.

When I first met the excellent Macmillan nurse (let's call her Petra, that being her name) who guided me through the early stages of diagnosis and treatment, one of the things that really surprised me (I nearly called this book *Cancer: a Surprising Journey*) was her response to my comment that she must be tired of constantly answering the many identical questions which all her clients must have. She told me that many of them don't ask *anything*. Several actually say they don't want to know any details. Tragically, not a few don't even get to the stage of meeting her at all: they get no further than their GP and never receive treatment. It is literally true that some people just don't want to know. I find this attitude very hard to fathom : Untreated, cancer kills. Treated, it usually doesn't. These are facts, and well-known ones too. The more facts we all know about cancer the better. There are symptoms which need to be acted on, there are foods and drink which must be avoided, there are tests you should take.

In any case, "I'm not going to think about it" is an impossible plan. If you have been diagnosed with cancer, you *cannot* not think about it. So you might as well think about it properly, researching as necessary and making decisions in the process. And then, getting on with the battle. It is, after all, *your* battle. All medicine does, in the end, it to help you fight. And the first and most important element to fighting is the determination to win. This is no idle talk: statistics show that those who feel involved in winning the battle against their cancer have better chances than those who do not. I'm sure you know of aged relatives who died soon after their spouses – just because they no longer wanted to live. Assuming you do want to, then act like it. Decide to get better, find out what you can, accept all the help you are offered and work with your medical team against the cancer.

Of course, there will be times (like when you've just been diagnosed) when it's not clear what the facts actually are. This is another important thing to be clear about, and well worth asking: how sure is the doctor about the facts, the treatment, the outcome? One of my most uplifting cancer-related experiences was meeting the surgeon who was going to remove my tumour. He said things like, "2% of people die in surgery in such cases", "1 in 5 patients show signs of nerve bruising" as well as "I don't know, there are insufficient data to answer that". I could have hugged the man. He was great. This is how I wanted to hear what I needed to know: clear, direct, accurate.

Finally, don't just ask the scary questions, make sure you understand the answers. Whatever those answers are, even if they may shock you at first, you will probably find they are less terrifying than you feared. There is always a way to improve your situation : there are always things that can help.

Another thing to bear in mind is that in a minority of cases, doctors may be reluctant to make things really clear in the case of a terminal prognosis. They are only human, they don't want too much upset in their day, and there is a natural temptation to not quite spell things out, to assume the patient gets the point. This is bad doctoring and if you come across it, you need to take charge: ask that hard question, and get a clear answer.

And... find out more. Read around. Go online (with care! There are brilliant websites around, but there are also a lot of blogs and other online material which has been out there by people with cancer. Inevitably, while such bloggers are often experts on their own kind of cancer, that may not be your kind and even if it is, their experiences, reactions and treatments many be very different. Also, there are plenty of bonkers people out there who believe in practically anything you can imagine, even homeopathy (the latter belief being bolstered by the inexplicable fact that some chemists stock the required bottle of very expensive, slightly impure, water)).

Now this may just be me, but knowing plenty about your state of health may make you feel that this whole cancer thing is actually handlable. Not very long ago, cancer was a mysterious killer, striking indiscriminately, almost invariably fatal. A dark and deadly menace lurking somewhere inside some of us, maybe even all of us. But, after just a little reading and discussion with experts, it soon becomes clear that cancer is largely understandable and treatable and just as much a part of life as everything else.

SIX You are going to die. But so is everyone else.

One day, you won't be here. Just as one day of the year is your birthday, another is the date on which you will die. If you're over fifty, you're probably more than halfway there already. You might, in fact, be dead tomorrow.

Why do I say what is obviously true? Because none of us believe it, that's why. We live our lives as if they are forever. We put things off for another day, confident that day will come and be followed by another and another in an endless stream. We overeat and overwork, we drink too much and don't exercise enough. We know that in so doing we are shortening our lives, but who cares about shortening something that feels like it will last forever?

Even when we do ponder how long we might have left, most of us are over-optimistic. The average life-expectancy of someone who is 65 in 2015, for example, is 12 years for a man, and 14 years for a woman. (But if you are 65, take heart! The average life-expectancy of someone born the same year you were is only 66 for males, 71 for females (the reason for the difference is the relatively high chance of dying within the first few months of life). Bear in mind too that you can easily beat the average by looking after your health). There is a table of life expectancies on page 69.

These mental approaches may well make us happier than facing the truth. But when the reality of our mortality is forced on us, by - for example – the diagnosis of terminal cancer, the sudden light of truth is shocking and may blind us to everything else. It feels like you've entered another world, but is it really so different to the old one? Perhaps you have 5 years left to live; it sounds terrible, but is about the same as that of an average 73-year old. Do all 73-year olds have lives of worry and fear? If not, why should you? I'm by no means trivializing the impact of being told your cancer cannot be eradicated, but it is the kind of news that almost everyone will one day receive. It is very natural to think "Why now?" "Why me?", but wouldn't you feel almost the same, whenever you heard such news?

SEVEN Expect the unexpected

"Expect the unexpected" can be an annoying phrase, but then the unexpected is a very annoying thing. But in the case of cancer, it not only makes sense to expect the unexpected, you can prepare for it too. For instance: at the numerous briefings, consultations, discussions and reviews building up to my operation, the question of a temporary stoma (see below) was vaguely aired, usually accompanied by some such phrase as "but don't worry about it", "it probably won't be needed", "we can discuss it closer to the time". Such phrases may be comforting, but they're not very helpful - or at least I didn't find them so.

A stoma, by the way, is a hole in an animal or person (plants breathe through them), and in bowel cancer treatment it's sometimes necessary to make one, by bringing a loop of gut to the surface. The loop is then cut, and the end of the bit leading to the anus is closed. The end of the other bit, that leads via the guts to the stomach, remains open on the surface of the body. Digested food (which is not quite poo yet; let's called it prepoo) passes out of this into a bag. I could go on at length about the wonders of stoma bags, their brilliant simplicity, ease of use and magical stickiness, which means that never fall off, yet don't irritate the skin they are stuck to and are easy to remove.... but I won't. The point is, I wanted to know all about this vague "temporary stoma" thing. What was it? Why might I need it? How long was "temporary" and - (a question guaranteed to make a large proportion of health workers look edgy), "What is the probability that I will need one?" So, with just a little reluctance, they told me all about it. As ever with common cancers and their treatment, there is oodles of information, guidance, self-help, phone numbers, images, diagrams and advice. I even got a pretend stoma complete with an artificial bit of gut sticking out of it, to practice on. It came complete with sachets to make pretend pseudo-pre-poo out of. It was almost fun.

Before the operation, one of the surgeons whom I spoke to thought it highly unlikely I'd need a stoma and the other (you do have a lot of conversations with experts when you have cancer!) was carefully neutral. When I woke up following the operation, guess what? There one was. Was I shocked? Or horrified? Not a bit of it. But I might have been, had I not "expected the unexpected."

As it was, since I had prepared I was OK. Not quite unbothered, but nonnonplussed. I had my information, I had my training, I even had a copy of a magazine called *Ostomy* and a blue bag kindly provided by the NHS to keep stoma-related paraphernalia in - I was ready to cope.

So, my point is ; always ask what might happen. Talk to the experts. Establish the possibilities. Estimate the probabilities. If the unexpected happens you'll be well prepared. If it doesn't, you'll have another thing to say, "well, it could have been worse" about.

EIGHT Diarise and memorise

One thing that cancer does is take over your diary. With chemotherapy in particular, it will map itself into your schedules for months in advance. This schedule may be helpfully diarised for you by your doctor or nurse, but that's just the main event - there will be lots of sideshows too. You will be handed a whole plethora of drugs, mostly to deal with side effects (so I hope you remembered that bag I mentioned in FIVE), and piles more information, including details of all sorts of support services.

Your diary is an ideal place to note what treatments and drugs you are given, and the people and places involved, too. You may be as astonished as I was at how many facts nurse and doctors think you will remember: Was it Estramustine Sodium Phosphate you had last time? Is it 250 ml you have? Which lotion was it we gave you? Which doctor told you that? Where did you have that done...?

The other thing worth noting down is instructions. It may sound very simple when the nurse says "take two of the red pills before breakfast and one yellow one after, then a white one at midday. And take two green ones if you feel sick". But when you are actually sitting there looking at a pile of boxes, it may not be so easy.

And then there are side effects: knowing just what, when, and how intense they are can be vital in helping your doctor plan future treatments. Correlating side effects with what you did (especially, what you ate), can really help avoid them too. So stick them in your diary. Not forgetting to then stick your diary in your pocket. Being over fifty, I still like paper diaries, but of course all the above could readily be done electronically.

It's also a good scheme to memorise people's names, as well as writing them down (in fact, writing them down may be enough in itself to remember them). Although all health workers do wear name badges, it's a bit of a giveaway if you have to peer at their chests or ever get your specs out before greeting them by name. They won't be surprised if you don't recall their name - but they will be pleased if you do.

Two tips that may help in remembering names are follows:

1. As soon as someone tells you their name, use it "Hi Mary, nice to meet you" "Hello John, what are you going to do with that syringe"... that kind of thing.
2. Associate the name with something. If someone is called Goulding, imagine something being gold-plated; for Smith imagine someone making a horseshoe. If they're called Ramsbottom... well, you get the idea.

NINE Don't take appointment times too seriously

One thing that infuriates everyone is to turn up for an appointment only to wait an hour, or to arrange to meet for dinner after a hospital visit, which turns out to overrun massively. However tempting it is (and it *is*) to blame someone, don't. It won't make you feel any better and it will only make the other person feel bad – and it's unlikely to be their fault. Almost always such problems really are unavoidable – the time a treatment will take can often only be roughly predicted, for instance. A fundamental problem is that there is such a large demand for appointments and treatments that there is no possibility of scheduling gaps between sessions to allow time lost by overrunning to be absorbed. So, usually, a delay to one appointment will often have a knock-on effect to all subsequent ones. But medical staff really do try to minimise this. When I was undergoing radiotherapy, I was more mobile than some other patients. Since there were several radiotherapy machines, I would often be allocated to first one, then another and occasionally even a third. This was because someone's treatment was taking longer than anticipated, thereby delaying all the people in the queue for that machine. If one of those later patients was me, I would be moved, if possible, to another machine which was not delayed. Balancing queues like this requires a oversight, organisation, communication and tact, and the staff tirelessly deployed those skills. This is all very well, you may be thinking, but it still leaves me hanging about in dull waiting rooms or missing appointments. Indeed it does, so don't just *wait* in waiting rooms - do something (see NINETEEN). And don't schedule anything until at least three hours after your appointment's planned end-time : you will only worry about missing it.

TEN Take someone with you....

Often, the first "proper" meeting with your oncologist passes in a blur, as you inevitably spend a lot of it thinking about cancer rather than concentrating on the many detailed things that are said – many of which involve words it's hard to imagine, let alone say or spell (personally I found Panitumumab a particular challenge). As a result, you may come out of the meeting feeling rather stunned and maybe not even clear what happens next. You may well also feel tearful, depressed, angry or shocked, with no ready outlet for those feelings. Even if you are calm and collected, it may still be hard to take things in during the meeting – especially if you have a long list of questions you want to ask, in which case there is the tendency to treat whatever the oncologist says as a stream of words you just want to end so you can start on your list. Finally, the oncologist may be wary of spelling things out, because (s)he is genuinely uncertain or because ... well, no-one likes upsetting people, do they? And there is also the very powerful influence of one 's own wishes. When the result of my first CT scan came back, the Macmillan nurse said something like, "The tumour looks quite small; there are some nearby lymph nodes that are enlarged, which might mean they are cancerous, but the swelling could be due to something else" What I heard was, "You're *fine!*" It was only when I relayed the message to a friend that I realised it was pretty likely that the nodes were cancerous. If I'd been thinking straight, I would have asked follow-up questions. As it was, just saying "great" to the nurse no doubt discouraged her from dragging me down again by discussing the swollen lymph nodes more, particularly since it was not certain what the cause of the swelling was. Why bother upsetting me, she probably thought, when things might be fine?

What does all this boil down to? That it's often a good plan to take to the meeting someone close to you, to comfort you and to remind you of what was said – or even to ask the specialist questions on your behalf if you feel too overwhelmed to do so.

ELEVEN ... or don't

The first few times I spoke to the excellent Macmillan nurse who explained and helped coordinate my care, she almost always reminded me that I could bring a partner or friends. Meanwhile, my partner and a number of close friends often suggested joining me.

And it was kind and right of them all to ask. But it was not what I wanted. I felt quite capable of listening and asking questions and quite confident of not breaking down in tears. You may be nothing like me (and in general I do think people prefer to take someone with them). But it may at least be worth asking yourself whether to want anyone to go with you or not : no-one will protest if you decline.

Assuming you *do* want someone with you, be sure you take the right person. Ask yourself: will they get very upset? Will (s)he be embarrassed if there are discussions about sex, or defecation? Will *I* be? Is (s)he the type that is likely to become impatient with waiting? Will (s)he keep talking afterwards when I want just to be quiet and think? And so on... There are no right answers here, so just visualise how the meeting will go with the person you are considering asking and take it from there.

TWELVE Conventional medicines work, alternatives don't

One of the many surprising things I learned by talking to a whole range of health workers, from surgeons to nurses to oncologists, is that some people really don't trust conventional medicine. In some cases the result is that they reject it in favour of alternatives. Which are really no alternatives at all: some may relieve some symptoms or help with relaxation, but none will tackle the root cause. If they did, the NHS would use them. And they do not.

A related issue is that some people are liable to reject offers of taking part in cancer trials that could help them. No-one will be worse off for taking the trials. There will be a control group who do not receive the trial drugs, but they do receive all the standard ones. That is not to say that every trial will be appropriate for everyone, but the oncologists and researchers involved in carrying them out will make certain that you are fully advised to make the best choice for yourself. They want to save your life, not to treat you as a guinea pig.

THIRTEEN Feelings from nowhere.

One day during your treatment, you may be sitting in a cafe with a friend and get a sudden rush of emotion, as is from nowhere. You may break down in tears, feel very depressed or react angrily to some innocent question. These emotions aren't irrational, they're simply delayed. When you receive any information you need time to process it, and with emotionally loaded news, this time can stretch into hours, days or even longer. (Judging by on-the-spot TV interviews, footballers seem especially plagued by the "it's not sunk in yet" reaction to their latest triumph/tragedy on the field, delaying the usual "over the moon"/"sick as a parrot" reaction). So, tragic news is numbing. But it's inevitable that those emotions *will* occur. Even after you have fully come to terms with the news, you will probably find that your feelings change rapidly from negative to positive and back again; you will sometimes feel really happy – honestly! When you do, don't tell yourself that your happiness is inappropriate or nonsensical – it isn't, and if it were, so what? Happy is good, so don't question it!

FOURTEEN Pets can be life-savers

Becoming a dog owner is one of the best decisions I ever made. Having a dog during cancer means you have someone who treats you the same as ever, still needs her exercise, her play, her training – everything. She's ecstatic to see you in the morning and happy to be stroked if you need affection. Other than avoiding being licked in the face, you should be able to play with your dog the same as ever. If you don't have one, visit someone who has.

Dogs are highly sensitive to the feelings of humans (a major reason for their great success in integrating with us) and you may well be surprised, as I was, that they will soon start taking your changed energy level or mood into account. My dog loves a tug of war, preceded by tempting me with the toy and followed by me throwing it for her. When she realised I was now too feeble to win the tugs of war, she would let me have the toy after a brief tussle. And later, when I had dizzy spells, she would be beside me the instant I sat down, wagging and licking and generally making things better.

I don't currently have a cat, but I know they are just as wonderful as dogs for people with, or recovering from, cancer. But it could be any pet really: a parrot, rabbit, horse; anyone you can interact with and love.

While on the subject: the short life spans of pets (other than tortoises and parrots) are realities which every pet owner has no choice but to get used to. And yet it rarely results in gloom. When I look at my dog and remember she will not be here in a dozen years, it encourages me to play with her, not to become despondent. And of course, she doesn't think about such prospects at all. That squeaky ball, that's what matters now.

Unlike those of animals, our minds are strangely predisposed to think about impending death (however far off) without ever actually coming to terms with it. But we can at least *try* to be more like dogs. We can live, however briefly, in the moment. And playing with a member of another species is an excellent way to starting thinking like one.

FIFTEEN There are things to enjoy

Cancer treatment needn't be unpleasant, especially once you are used to the routine. Chemotherapy and radiotherapy appointments are often made at the same times each week, which means that the days on which you feel at your best will probably be quite predictable. On those days, you may well be able to do most of the things you want to. Days when you don't feel up to do any more than sitting on the sofa need not be wasted either: why not read one of those books you always meant to? Or explore the world of film? Personally, I splashed out on a magic pair of electric goggles that mean I have a whole 3D movie theatre going on an inch from my head.

There are ways to make the best of other effects of cancer or its treatment. My skin became sensitive to bright sunlight, so I started wearing hats - which turned out to look rather cool, if I do say so myself. Another consequence of the chemotherapy was that I lost weight - no bad thing in itself, and it also meant I could eat as much as I felt like for a change. It may need a bit of thought, research or discussion, but finding ways to enjoy some aspects of your changed life can make a huge difference.

Then again, you may have an interest in a subject which your treatment - and the free time it gives you - will allow you to explore. I'm a scientist, which meant I had an *excellent* time in the radiotherapy unit of Charing Cross Hospital, which is packed with the most amazing technology, plus loads of people who love to enthuse about it (though admittedly rather pressed for time). X rays and electrons zapping about, vast magnetic fields under precise control, imaging software that makes your eyes water (in a good way). Lovely stuff. If science isn't your thing, well, that particular hospital also contains lots of historical material about nursing, shedloads of contemporary and classic artworks on display - and even some resident eagles on its roof. And of course hospitals are full of people, some of whom are bound to share your interests. One of the oncologists whom I saw regularly was fascinated by the way the brain relates to the mind, and so am I, so we talked about that as often as about cancer, and swapped book suggestions too. Support groups, like those offered by Maggie's, offer yet more opportunities to follow up interests.

SIXTEEN Talk to your support team

Your hospital is likely to become very familiar to you during your treatment. So it makes sense to know both how it works and what it offers - is there more than one place to go for your blood tests? Which lifts are quicker? Are some days/times of day better than others for parking? Is there a library? A Bookshop? Where is Clinical Imaging? When does the cafe close? And so on. Just ask; hospitals are packed with helpful, patient and knowledgeable people happy to help.

Among the huge range of excellent services to which you will have access, from home visits to charity-based activities, to the many kinds of therapies and tests, don't forget your GP. (S)he will be kept informed of your progress by your oncologist and other specialists, and will be more familiar than they are with your medical history and probably your personality too. (S)he will be nearer than your hospital too and might well be the easiest expert to see at short notice (GPs often have an informal "fast track" service for patients with cancer). You may also find it easier to talk to him/her about some of the effects of cancer, perhaps related to sex, anxiety or digestion. And, so that you don't have to pay for your prescriptions (s)he'll sort you out a Medical Exemption Certificate too.

SEVENTEEN Ways of escape

One thing about cancer is that it and its treatments will become a major part of your life for months or years. Your diary will fill with appointments, your bathroom cabinet with medicines and your mind with new information. Some things you used to do may become impossible, or must be reduced or modified. (But make sure they really *must*. A fellow sufferer, David, had a stoma bag, as I do. Whenever we talked about what he was doing or would like to do, the bag popped up (not literally). It seemed like some over-protective companion who prevented him from doing *anything*. Going on holiday. Having a bath. Having a shower. Crawling about in the undergrowth where greater spotted woodpeckers lurked. Eating his favourite things. Sleeping. Well, maybe it did – but I did all those things very successfully with mine. Even the undergrowth thing. (Though not because I'm a bird watcher: my dog specialises in finding lost footballs deeply embedded in nettles and thistles, invisible to all but the doggy eye but sadly irretrievable by canine kind. Her retrieval technique is 1. Sit staring at the ball. 2. Glance at me in a confident manner. 3. Adopt a tragic look and, if I'm still not really trying, 4. whine quietly.) The joy with which she greets the ball far outweighs the additions to my collection of stings and scratches and the missing bits of my latest woolly jumper. But, as they say in old books, I digress...).

Having decided what you *really* can't do, you may very well, and very naturally, not be happy with the result. You didn't ask for this, you don't deserve it. But you *can* escape it : the modern world offers an unprecedented wealth of methods to experience, learn and enjoy things without moving from your comfy sofa. The vast accumulation of knowledge and entertainment that has been built up over centuries, from books to artworks to music to films to games is, quite suddenly, now just a mouse click away – often for free.

If any aspect of this sounds a bit daunting, just remember that vast queue of people who offered to help in any way they could (in TWO). It's a fair bet that some of them are absolute wizards at selecting, loads, using and demonstrating a Kindle. If they're really into it, they probably have numerous old versions knocking about just waiting for a home. With you!

Even better than something passive like book reading or film-watching, is something constructive/creative/useful – again, the internet is a great help here. Writing is an obvious one (well, it is to me, anyway), but there's also programming, composition, researching, cartooning, editing your old photos, sorting out your family tree – the world's your oyster (whatever that means).

EIGHTEEN On waiting

Waiting. There's a lot of it about when you've got cancer. Strangely, people seem to treat it as a different sort of waiting to the kind they do on, say, a train. There, they chat, read, text, play online games, listen to music, work... constructive, creative, even enjoyable waiting. But waiting for tests, results, consultations or treatments is very different. Usually, people just... well, sit there, sometimes for hours. Is this because they are bowed down by pain or misery or fear? Of course some are, and others are too ill to do anything other than nothing. But many are not. For some, this doing-nothing-ness seems to be an aspect of switching-off of all involvement in their treatment. Doctors and nurses and would come and ask things and the person would answer – but with no engagement, no follow-up questions.

As well as hanging about in waiting rooms, cancer also involves a lot of waiting for days or weeks for results, appointments or treatments. To deal with this, try involving yourself deeply in some activity, ideally one which tires the body and engages the mind too. If you find yourself getting into a panic, or a rage, about waiting, it might help to remind yourself that really a few days or weeks here or there will make no difference. Of course, it makes no sense to tell yourself an couple of hours' delay doesn't matter if in fact it does. The moral being: don't schedule anything else just after the end of your appointment-time. During my chemotherapy, for many reasons, end times were fairly unpredictable. Since I always had something do during the therapy and nothing to do straight afterwards, that didn't matter – except the one time I'd arranged to be collected at a particular time - that was *really* stressful!

Always ask how long you might have to wait for. You may find that some health workers tend to err on the side of optimism, perhaps to avoid upsetting you but also because they may be embarrassed that things don't move faster. It's worth discussing the question a little - how often are such things delayed? What causes the delays? If there is a delay next visit, is it likely to be a last minute one, or would ringing ahead be a good idea? In this way you can avoid being taken by surprise by delays, which usually makes them less upsetting. Bear in mind though that the person you talk to might take your questions as criticisms or doubts, so make it clear from your tone and wording that you're not complaining.

When you know how long your wait will be, you can plan around it. These days, hospitals are often well provided with things like bookshops and coffee bars, and if there is a Maggie's Centre attached (or something similar - West Middlesex Hospital has a brilliant charitable support centre called the Mulberry, for instance), a long delay can be an ideal opportunity to explore. Let the receptionist know where you are going though, and leave them your mobile number, just in case things move unexpectedly quickly.

NINETEEN Naps conquer all

In around 1600 Shakespeare, who is always an excellent chap when one is in search of a few words of wisdom expressed in beautiful language, said,

... the innocent sleep,
Sleep that knits up the ravell'd sleave of care,
The death of each day's life, sore labour's bath,
Balm of hurt minds, great nature's second course,
Chief nourisher in life's feast.

And quite right he was too. There's nothing like a nap – and, during treatment, you're likely to be tired quite often. Naps are especially useful if you're having trouble sleeping at night, and it's been shown that even short ones during the day can make up for the effect of several lost hours at night. The only problem with naps is that, if you're exhausted, you may find they can turn easily into deep sleep, from which it's difficult to wake and after which you may feel lousy - to avoid this, it may help to doze off in a chair rather than lying down. If you find it difficult to stop thinking, try watching an old film or listening to music (with the sound low). Concentrate on that and you'll soon find yourself dropping off. A hot milky drink can also help a lot.

TWENTY Push your limits – gently

One very common effect of cancer treatments is weariness. While it may be tempting to give in to this and stay indoors without much moving around, it's a bad idea to make this a habit. There are diseases for which bed rest is essential but cancer is not one of them. For your body to fight it, it needs to be fairly fit and active, and exercise helps this process, Your body is engaged in civil war, and the good guys need to be fit and focussed: lots of bright red blood cells surging about, a well-functioning digestive system providing nourishment, a lymphatic system busily clearing out the rubbish, lungs supplying all the oxygen your cells need to grow and prosper. And all of these systems suffer if you laze about. Exercise is also likely to alleviate, at least to some extent, the feeling of depression that cancer can so easily generate. How much exercise depends very much on what you are used to and how you are feeling. If your pre-cancer activities were mainly limited to walking to the car, or if you feel really shattered by the treatment, a short walk a couple of times a day will be enough to work wonders. It's a good idea to take a friend, especially for your first few outings, just in case they are a bit more than you can handle. It will take time to know what you can cope with (and also, at least in my experience, the tiredness associated with cancer treatment is the sort that creeps up and pounces: often I would start an one hour dog-walk quite comfortably, but feel a sudden need for rest after 20 minutes or so. In my case, sitting on a handy bench made me feel a lot better, fast). If you do find you get suddenly tired, rest and/or return and make a mental (or written) note of when that point was reached. There's no particular need to push your limits : if 10 minutes a day is enough for you, there's no reason to force yourself to do 20. On the other hand, it is worth just nudging those limits gently from time to time, maybe adding a few minutes to your walk every few days. The reason for nudging limits is that you will (honestly!) start to feel better after a while, and you may find yourself quite able to do some extra minutes. People often say about such situations "listen to your body", and this is right in a way, but the trouble it that behaviours tend to reinforce themselves, so just as you can get used to a sticky cake each day you don't really need, so you can get used to lazing about on the sofa when you could just as easily be leaping about the hills.

But don't fool yourself - though walking is much better than nothing, something even more exerting is better still: like swimming, cycling or running. Again, don't push yourself more than a little, if the exercise makes you out of breath, and/or your muscles ache pleasantly a few hours later, it's doing you good. Again, going with a friend is a good plan.

TWENTY-ONE Get outdoors

There will be days – maybe a handful, maybe a majority – when you feel like doing nothing whatsoever and end up lying on the sofa deteriorating. You may have been told, as I was, that it's fine to feel low. Fine to be gloomy, to complain, to cry, to feel despondent. If you ask me, that's rubbish. Giving in is not fine. It *might* sometimes be unavoidable, but it should be fought, especially if it becomes a habit. One simple thing which works for almost everyone, at least to some extent, is simply going outdoors, ideally somewhere with trees. The garden is good, a park is better and the countryside is best of all. Ring up one of those people who offered to help (in TWO) and get them to go with you if you like, call a taxi, jump on a train, but get out there. So what if it's raining? You don't have to walk far, or fast, or stay out for long. If you feel at all uncertain about venturing out alone, then of course go with someone else, but if you do, just make sure they are fully aware of your limits. Make it clear that you're not going out to get fit, lose weight, or anything else, other than to be outside (of course, if you like, you can easily combine these outings with the exercise activities mentioned in TWENTY). Once you're there, don't stomp along with your eyes on the ground, thinking. Look around. See things. If you're so inclined, take a map or a book of walks or a wildlife guide(or online versions of such things). And, plan a visit to a cafe, pub, castle, church or museum during or after your walk too.

TWENTY-TWO Is it a journey?

I don't know about you, but I have a very low threshold when it comes to posters of cute animals announcing trite pleasantries like "life goes better with a smile" One such phrase, however, does strike me as very true, which is "cancer is a journey". For one thing, treatment seems to go on for bloody ever, like some kind of endless world cruise. For another, cancer is a whole series of new experiences – and not all nasty ones by any means (see FIFTEEN) But perhaps the most telling similarity is the way that, like a really good journey, the cancer experience will tell you about yourself. But there are many sorts of journeys, and cancer is not the kind where you can lay back and wait for nice things to happen. It's more like a hiking trip: effort and exertion is required, there will be false starts, sticky patches, thistles and mud. But there will be progress, hurdles overcome, many small triumphs and - mostly - a clear route forward.

TWENTY-THREE Your cancer is not you

You might sometimes feel that you are regarded by health workers as a collection of cancer symptoms, rather than a person. But it's unlikely that they really feel like this about you (they would probably never have gone for the job unless they were genuinely caring people). And don't be tempted to think of yourself like that either: because cancer is a long-term condition, it's vital that you play an active role in the battle: it's you versus the disease, with health workers assisting you. On the other hand, though beating your cancer is probably going to be your top priority for months, that doesn't mean cancer is all your life is; see FOURTEEN, FIFTEEN, and SEVENTEEN.

TWENTY-FOUR Be part of the solution

For the reasons given in NINE, delays are an inevitable part of treatment and though the (five!) hospitals and clinics I attended during my treatment had planning and booking systems which reduced them as far as possible. Sometimes, however, you may spot genuine daftnesses in the systems of which you are a part, or problems to which there is an obvious solution. Perhaps you find it hard to work out where you are supposed to be, or can't hear loudspeaker announcements. Maybe you often find the drinking water has run out, or can't stand the background music. In cases like this, you can be pretty sure that you are not the only one who is bothered – so, speak out (or, if you'd rather remain anonymous, seek out the nearest Suggestion Box). It's quite possible that hospital staff genuinely don't know there is a problem and may well be able to remedy it.

TWENTY-FIVE Have things to look forward to

Most cancers and their treatments have major impacts on many aspects of life, including work, sports and holidays. Some of the changes that result are unavoidable, like rescheduling things around therapy dates. Others are less clear-cut. You may feel exhausted, but still able to force yourself to go to work, or to keep up regular swimming, say. In such cases, make sure you ask your oncologist whether it is actually safe for you to go on working or swimming. If it is, and if there is no practical reason for you to stop, then have a serious think about whether to continue or not. This depends very much on your personality – it may be really important to your sense of self-worth to keep going, or you may be sure that running or working is the best way to keep yourself from worrying. In this particular case, conversations with partners, family or friends may be counter-productive: even people who know you way may be inclined to give unsuitable advice, like "take the time off, no-one will blame you and you've earned it"- which may be true, but does not take account of the fact that you may really want to keep working.

Whatever changes are forced on you, or that you decide to make, it's important to arrange non cancer-related things to do, ideally small simple things that can be rescheduled if necessary. Not only will doing these things help occupy you, the activity of planning them should make you feel more in control – and make your life fuller too. Your diary will inevitably start to fill with cancer-related appointments, but there's no reason not to fill it even further with fun things.

If you're sure what those things might be - or can't imagine anything being fun – find out about what cancer charities in your hospital or area have on offer. You'll probably be surprised at how much they have for you to do (and it's almost always free).

But don't become too attached to those things. Cancer often has a trick up its sleeve and it's possible you may - for example - develop an infection, or have a low blood count, or be laid low by some side effect, which means that you have to modify your plans. So, always have a back-up version: if you can't go to the theatre to see a play, maybe it's on DVD. If going to the South of France has to be put on hold, how about the Lake District? Can't make it to Skye to see your friend – ideal time to get into Skype. And so on.

TWENTY-SIX Get over it – and keep those good habits

When treatment ends, it's hard to believe it really has. After months of appointments, discussions, treatments, tests and forms, all becomes quiet, except for regular check-up appointments. Usually, these go on for five years, and to begin with they are most often 3-monthly. As you by now have become so used to focussing on the next appointment, there is a natural tendency to do the same now, and count down the days to that check-up. Don't do it. Cancer has already taken months of your life, and you've had no choice about that. Now you *do* have a choice, to live a normal life or to continue thinking of yourself as a patient. You're not. Just like your 6-monthly dental check-up, your annual set of cholesterol tests, or your two-yearly eye test, your next check-up is something you should not think about on an hourly, daily or even weekly basis. "Ah, but", you may think, "this is different. They might tell me I've got cancer again." Yes, they might. If they do, this three months beforehand is going to be the only time you're free of cancer for while – so why not enjoy them?

TWENTY-SEVEN Give something back

You may feel extremely put-upon and generally got-at for having cancer and unhappy that you are unable to do the things you used to do, spend hours being treated, and so on. But you may also feel grateful to the NHS, to medical science, or to the people who looked after you in hospital. If you do, you might consider giving something back. This need not take the form of a charitable contribution, though these are vital to the continued provision of many support services (there's a list of major cancer charities on page 65). Volunteers have a major role in cancer treatment, and do things like fetching drugs, assisting at drop-in centres, providing expertise for free (perhaps regarding legal issues, financial matters or exercise suggestions). Talk to your GP, hospital, Maggie's Centre or any other charity if you think you might want to do this.

A very different way to give something back - which might just give something back to you in turn - is to volunteer to take part in a clinical trial. As mentioned in TWELVE, getting involved in one is completely risk-free. While some involve new drugs, these drugs have all been thoroughly safety-tested first, so there is really no good reason not to take part. There are literally thousands of trials, for all kinds of cancer, and for all kinds of patients. Without these trials, the amazing progress in cancer treatment over the last few decades would not have happened. The weblinks on page 49 include one to the UK trials database.

TWENTY-EIGHT It can take longer to free the mind of cancer than the body

Cancer is insidious. Long after treatment ends, it lurks in the mind. Partly, this is because there is never a time when you can be absolutely certain it will not return. But also, cancer reminds you you are mortal. So, just acknowledge that is true and decide to make the most of the time that remains.

TWENTY-NINE Cancer's not fair. Which can help.

Cancer, just like most diseases, is unpredictable. Statistics are just collections of facts from the past and the fact that only 5% of people in your situation die from their cancer does not mean that you will not. But remember that the reverse is also true – though 95% of people may die from the sort of cancer you have, you may not. Chance can work for you, just as much as it can work against you: in 2011, an eight-year old girl called Claudia Burkhill was diagnosed with a rare kind of brain cancer, one for which the probable life-span was a few days. Three years later she was completely cancer free, thanks to very high-dose chemo and radio-therapy, and a lot of good luck. There are also cases of "super-responders", for whom anti-cancer drugs work with almost incredible effectiveness. Super-responders are rare and lucky- but that doesn't mean you're not one of them.

THIRTY Watch out

After your treatment has ended, it is time to put cancer behind you and return to all those things that cancer postponed, and do all those things you decided to do during your treatment: see friends, go on holiday, smell the roses, train the dog to shut the door. Don't waste your time worrying that your cancer will return; all you need to do is be aware of warning signs, as everyone should be anyway. See page 56 for a list of things to watch out for.

FINALLY...

I hope that the ideas in this book have been of some help, or at least of interest. They are only my opinions of course, based on my own experiences: and neither all cancers nor all experiences of cancer will be the same. Whether this book has been of help or not, you may like to read others and the Further Reading section contains some suggestions. There's a separate section for recommended books about specific cancers. I've also included sections containing basic factual information - to find out more, try the weblinks on the next page...

If you have any tips you'd like to be included in the next edition, or any comments about this book, please drop me a line at 30thingsabout@gmail.com

Good luck!

Weblinks

Cancer information – NHS Choices
http://www.nhs.uk/conditions/cancer/Pages/Introduction.aspx

Cancer Research UK
http://www.cancerresearchuk.org

Clinical trials
http://www.cancerresearchuk.org/about-cancer/trials/trials-search/

Glossary
http://www.cancerresearchuk.org/about-cancer/utilities/glossary

Macmillan Cancer Support
http://www.macmillan.org.uk

Maggie's centres
https://www.maggiescentres.org/

Marie Curie Cancer Care
https://www.mariecurie.org.uk

Statistics
http://www.ncbi.nlm.nih.gov/pubmed/25479696
http://www.thelancet.com/journals/lancet/article/PIIS0140-6736%2814%2961396-9/abstract

Further Reading : General

Mind Over Mood: Change How You Feel By Changing the Way You Think, Aaron T Beck and Dennis Greenberger, 2010

There's Something I've Been Dying to Tell You, Lynda Bellingham, 2014

The Feeling Good Handbook, David D Burns, 1999

Positive: Finding Life in the Midst of Cancer, Sally Collings, 2009

Sweet Sorrow: Love, Loss and Attachment in Human Life, Alan B. Eppel, 2009

Being Mortal: Illness, Medicine and What Matters in the End, Atul Gawande, 2014

Secrets of Cancer Survivors, Elizabeth Gould, 2008

Added Time: Surviving Cancer, Death Threats and the Premier League, Mark Halsey and Ian Ridley, 2013

Please Don't Go: Big John's Journey Back to Life, John Hartson, 2007

Overcoming Anxiety, Helen Kennerley, 2014

Coming to Terms with Cancer : A Glossary of Cancer-Related Terms Easily Understood, Edward H. Laughlin, 2013

The C-Word, Lisa Lynch, 2010

How To Help Yourself While on Chemotherapy, Natalie Mitchell, 2016

The Emperor of All Maladies: A Biography of Cancer, Siddhartha Mukherjee, 2011

What to do when they say it's Cancer, Joel Nathan, 1998

Nine Lives: A Story of Survival and Hope: Overcoming Obstacles, Labels and Beating the Odds, Paul Nemiroff and Brian Solon, 2014

Worms on Parachutes: Mystical Allies in My Cancer Survival, Sarah-Jane Phillips, 2013

Cancer Fitness: Exercise Programs For Patients And Survivors, Anna L. Schwartz, 2004

Cancer at your Fingertips, Val Speechley, 2001

This is Living!: The Joys of Illness, Marea Stenmark, 2014

The Total Cancer Wellness Guide, Kim Thiboldeaux and Mitch Golant, 2007

100 Questions and Answers about Life After Cancer, Page Tolbert and Penny Damaskos, 2007

To give to friends and family

Caring for Someone with Cancer, Toni Battison, 2003

What Can I Do to Help?: 75 Practical Ideas for Family and Friends from Cancer's Frontline, Deborah Hutton, 2010

What Not to Say to a Cancer Patient: How to Talk about Cancer and Create a Supportive Network Paperback, Paul L. Bishop, 2013

Further Reading : Specific Cancers

BLADDER

100 Questions and Answers About Bladder Cancer, Pamela Ellsworth, 2006

BOWEL / COLON / RECTAL

Beating Bowel Cancer, Tim Darvell and Joanna Rubery, 2012

Your Guide to Bowel Cancer, John Northover, 2007

Coping with Bowel Cancer, Tom Smith, 2005

BRAIN

Brain Tumours: Living low grade, Gideon Burrows, 2013

Brain Tumors: Leaving the Garden of Eden - A Survival Guide to Diagnosis, Learning the Basics, Getting Organized and Finding Your Medical Team, Paul M. Zeltzer, 2004

BREAST

Breast Cancer : Taking Control, John Boyages, 2010

B is for Breast Cancer: From anxiety to recovery and everything in between - a beginner's guide, Christine Hamill, 2014

Navigating Breast Cancer, A Guide for the Newly Diagnosed, Lillie Shockney, 2007.

CERVICAL

100 Questions and Answers About Cervical Cancer, Don S. Dizon, 2009

COLON - SEE BOWEL

ESOPHAGEAL
100 Questions and Answers about Esophageal Cancer, Pamela Ginex, 2005

GASTRIC - SEE STOMACH

HEAD AND NECK
100 questions and Answers About Head and Neck Cancer, Elise Carper, 2008.

LEUKAEMIA / LYMPHOMA / MYELOMA

Living with Leukaemia, Lymphoma and Myeloma :a Guide for Patients and Their Families, Pam McGrath, 2008

LIVER

100 Questions and Answers About Liver Cancer, Ghassan K. Alfa, 2006

LUNG

ABC of Lung Cancer, Ian Hunt, 2008

How to Survive Lung Cancer - A Practical 12-Step Plan, Michael Lloyd, 2007

100 Questions and Answers About Lung Cancer, Karen Parles, 2009

MELANOMA - SEE SKIN

MESOTHELIOMA - SEE SKIN

ORAL

Meeting the Challenges of Oral and Head and Neck Cancer: A Guide for Survivors and Caregivers, Nancy E. Leupold and James Sciubba, 2011

OVARIAN

100 Questions and Answers About Ovarian Cancer, Don S. Dizon and Nadeem R. Abu-Rustum, 2007

PANCREATIC

100 Questions and Answers About Pancreatic Cancer, Eileen O'Reilly, 2010

PROSTATE

Prostate Cancer for Dummies, Paul H. Lange, 2003

Prostate Cancer: Understand, Prevent and Overcome, Jane A. Plant, 2004

Prostate Cancer (The Facts), Malcolm Mason and Leslie Moffat, 2010

RECTAL - SEE BOWEL

SKIN / MESOTHELIOMA / MELANOMA

Fast Facts: Skin Cancer, Karen L. Agnew and Barbara A. Gilchrest, 2005

100 Questions and Answers About Mesothelioma, Harvey Pass, 2005.

STOMACH / GASTRIC

100 Questions and Answers About Gastric Cancer, Manish A Shah, 2008

TESTICULAR

Testicular Cancer - The Essential Guide, Priya Shah, 2013

THYROID

The Complete Thyroid Book, Kenneth B. Ain, 2005

UTERINE

Uterine Cancer (100 Questions & Answers), Don S. Dizon, 2010

Warning signs

Go to your GP if you experience any of these:

Change in bowel or bladder habits

Sore that does not heal

Unusual bleeding or discharge

Lump in the breast, testicles, or elsewhere

Persistent or frequent indigestion, cough or hoarseness

Difficulty swallowing

Obvious change in the size, colour, shape, or thickness of a wart, mole, or
mouth sore

Less reliable signs (these may have causes other than cancer, but are still likely to be serious, so go to your GP if you have any of them)

- Persistent headaches
- Unexplained loss of weight or loss of appetite
- Chronic pain in bones or any other areas of the body
- Persistent fatigue, nausea, or vomiting
- Persistent low-grade fever, either constant or intermittent
- Repeated infection

Causes

Most cancers happen when there are two of more of these causes working together.

Age
The risk of getting most cancers increases with age.

Cancer causing substances (carcinogens)
Tobacco is a major cause of lung cancer and can also cause oral cancer.

Environment
Sunlight can cause skin cancer, radiation can cause a wide range of cancers.

Genetics
Some people are born with a greater chance of getting some cancers, including breast and bowel cancer.

Weakened immune system
Due to treatment with immunosuppresant drugs (following organ transplant, for example), or to having HIV or AIDS.

Lifestyle
Smoking, being overweight, excessive drinking, eating a lot of processed food or not eating enough fresh fruit and vegetables all increase the risks of getting a wide range of cancers.

Viruses

Though cancer is not caused by a virus (and is not infectious), there are some viruses which make particular cancers more likely: the human papilloma virus (HPV) makes people more vulnerable to cervical cancer; hepatitis B and C make liver cancer more likely, the Epstein-Barr virus increases the risk of lymphomas and infection by the Human T cell leukaemia virus can be followed by T cell leukaemia.

Bacteria

Having a helicobacter pylori (H pylori) stomach infection increases the risk of stomach cancer.

Scans

Very often, in order to diagnose your cancer, find out more about it, or check that treatment is working, your oncologist will arrange for you to be scanned. In some cases this will involve a part of your body, such as your abdomen, while in others a whole-body scan will be carried out. Scanning involves detecting radiation from your body and then using a computer to generate images of your organs from the detections. There are three main types. Usually, the procedure is the same: you lie on a soft platform which moves you into a tube-shaped machine which contains the scanning equipment. Scanning usually takes between ten minutes and half an hour, though in a few cases it can take up to 90 minutes. You will have to keep still during the process. If your chest is being scanned, you may need to hold your breath for a few seconds (though some machines automatically detect your breathing rhythm and correct for it). If your abdomen is being scanned you may be given water to drink just before the scan, so that the bladder is full and pushes the organs around it out, making them easier to see. Sometimes a small tube called a cannula (from the Latin word for "little reed") will be positioned in your arm and liquid fed into your bloodstream through this. The liquid is a contrast agent, which is very easy for the machine to detect, so that a clear image of your blood vessels and other organs can be produced. You will often be asked not to eat for a few hours before a scan. You will usually need to remove some of your clothes, and wear a hospital gown.

CT (Computed Tomography) scan
A CT scan (which used to be called a CAT scan) uses X-rays to image the interior of your body. Unlike X-rays you might have to check your teeth, CT scans can detect soft tissues as well as bones and teeth. As well as CT machines which are used just to look inside you, there are some which are built into radiotherapy machines, which are used to aim the radiotherapy beam accurately.

MRI (Magnetic Resonance Imaging) scan

An MRI scan involves the detection of radio waves rather than X-rays. The process involves generating an extremely powerful magnetic field in your body, and then switching it off. A burst of radio waves is produced by your tissues at this point, and these are detected and used to build images of your organs. The machine is very similar in appearance to a CT machine but it is much noisier, so you will be given headphones or earplugs to wear.

Ultrasound scan

Ultrasound machines are much smaller and simpler than CT, MRI or PET machines. They consist of a combined loudspeaker and microphone, which sends sound waves into your body, and detects then when they come out again. Changes in the waves allow a computer to build up an image of the area. Some ultrasound devices are small enough to be inserted into your body briefly, to make even closer scans of some organs (such as the ovaries or the prostate)

PET (Positron Emission Spectroscopy) scan

While CT, MRI and ultrasound scans provide images of your organs, PET scans highlight areas of rapid cell division. Since cancer cells divide rapidly, they can be detected in this way, so a PET scan can be used to check whether a structure that looks suspicious is actually cancerous or not. Before the scan is made, you will be injected with glucose which is slightly radioactive. Cells which are dividing rapidly need more fuel than others, and glucose is one of these fuels. So, the glucose becomes concentrated in cancerous tissue. The radiation (gamma rays) that it produces are detected by the machine. You will remain radioactive for a few hours after the procedure, which is harmless to yourself and other adults but you will be asked to keep away from babies or pregnant women, and you should also avoid puppies and other young pets if you have them.

How the stages of cancer are defined

In the UK, two different systems are used to describe the way cancer develops. When you are diagnosed with cancer, it will be "staged", that is, your oncologist will work out how advanced the cancer is. Blood cancers like leukaemia and lymphomas have different systems, but for the other cancer types, the systems are:

TNM staging

TNM is short for Tumour, Node, Metastasis. TNM staging describes the size of the Tumour, how many lymph Nodes it has spread to, if any, and whether it has spread ("Metastasised") to other organs.

T may be 1, 2, 3, or 4. 1 is the smallest.

N ranges from 0 (no lymph nodes contain cancer cells) to 3 (many lymph nodes contain cancer cells)

M is either 0 (the cancer hasn't spread to any other organs) or 1 (it has)

(The lymph nodes are part of the lymphatic system, which is a network of thin tubes that run throughout the body and helps fight infections. Lymph nodes also trap cancer cells).

Staging by numbers

Stage 1 (I) : only one organ contains cancer cells, and the tumour is small.

Stage 2 (II) : the tumour is larger. In some cancers (including breast and lung), stage 2 can mean the cancer has spread into nearby lymph nodes. In others, including bowel cancer, stage 2 means the cancer has not spread into nearby lymph node.

Stage 3 (III) : there are cancer cells in nearby lymph nodes, and sometimes in other nearby tissues.

Stage 4 (IV) : the cancer has spread ("metastasised") to at least one other organ.

Treatments

There are three main cancer treatments:

Surgery
As well as being used to remove cancer, surgery can be used to take samples (biopsies) in order to confirm cancer is present or to find out more about it.

Chemotherapy
Chemotherapy involves the use of drugs to kill cancer. There are more than fifty such drugs, often used in combination. Sometimes they are taken as pills, sometimes fed directly into a vein, in hospital. Chemotherapy is often used alongside radiotherapy, to make cancer cells more vulnerable to radiation.

Radiotherapy
Radiotherapy is the use of high energy rays to destroy cancer cells. Usually the rays come from a machine, but sometimes radioactive substances are implanted temporarily into the body (brachytherapy). Radiotherapy is also sometimes used to deal with cancer symptoms.

Other treatments

Biological therapies : using antibodies, vaccines or genetics.

Hormone therapies : taking control of the body's own hormones to destroy cancer cells.

Photodynamic therapy (PDT): using chemicals that make cancer cells sensitive to light, which is then used to destroy them.

Radiofrequency ablation: radio waves are used to heat a metal fibre which is positioned close to cancer cells. They are killed by the heat.

Transplants : of stem cells or bone marrow.

Major charities

Cancer Research UK

Cancer Research UK is the world's largest cancer research charity. It researches the prevention, diagnosis and treatment of the disease, partly by funding researchers in universities and hospitals. It also provides information about cancer.

http://www.cancerresearchuk.org

Macmillan Cancer Support

Macmillan Cancer Support provides specialist health care, information and financial support to people affected by cancer.

As well as helping with the medical needs of people affected by cancer, Macmillan also looks at the social, emotional and practical impact cancer can have, and campaigns for better cancer care. Macmillan Cancer Support's goal is to reach and improve the lives of everyone living with cancer in the UK.

The charity was founded, as the Society for the Prevention and Relief of Cancer, in 1911 by Douglas Macmillan following the death of his father from the disease.

http://www.macmillan.org.uk

Maggie's

Maggie's centres provide free practical, emotional and social support to people with cancer and their family and friends, following the ideas about cancer care proposed by Maggie Keswick Jencks.

Built in the grounds of NHS cancer hospitals, Maggie's Centres are places with professional staff on hand to offer the support people need.

The first Maggie's Centre opened in Edinburgh in 1996

Locations
Aberdeen : Aberdeen Royal Infirmary
Cheltenham : Cheltenham General Hospital
Dundee : Ninewells Hospital
Edinburgh : Western General Hospital
Fife : Victoria Hospital
Glasgow : Western Infirmary
Hong Kong : Tuen Mun Hospital
Inverness : Raigmore Hospital
Lanarkshire : Monklands Hospital, Airdrie
London : Charing Cross Hospital
Merseyside : Clatterbridge Cancer Centre
Newcastle : Freeman Hospital
Nottingham : City Hospital
Oxford : Churchill Hospital
Swansea : Singleton Hospital

https://www.maggiescentres.org/

Marie Curie Cancer Care

Marie Curie Cancer Care is a charity that provides free nursing care, to terminally ill people at home and in hospices. It was established in 1948.

https://www.mariecurie.org.uk

Facts and stats

Definition of cancer

"Cancer is when abnormal cells divide in an uncontrolled way. Some cancers may eventually spread into other tissues. Cancer starts when gene changes make one cell or a few cells begin to grow and multiply too much. This may cause a growth called a tumour."

One in two people born after 1960 in the UK will be diagnosed with some form of cancer during their lifetime.

50% of adult cancer patients diagnosed in 2010-2011 in England and Wales are predicted to survive 10 or more years.

Cancer survival in the UK has doubled in the last 40 years.

There are more than 200 different types of cancer. Cancer can develop cancer in any of the body's organs.

The three most common cancers in men
1. Prostate
2. Lung
3. Bowel

The three most common cancers in women
1. Breast
2. Lung
3. Bowel

(all data from Cancer Research UK)

Commonness of cancer as cause of death in the USA
1910 8th
1960 2nd
2014 2nd

Source
http://www.businessinsider.com/leading-causes-of-death-from-1900-2010-2012-6?op=1&IR=T

Mean survival rates for all cancers in the UK
1971   1 year
1980   1½years
1990   2 years
2000   4 years
2007   6 years

(note: these figures do not mean that most people who got cancer in 2007 survived for 6 years; these numbers are averages: many people who got cancer in 2000, for instance, are still alive today, while many others died within a year or two. The reason that it is average survival times that are given, rather than the number of people cured, is that it is hard to decide when cancer has been cured. Usually, if cancer does return, it will happen within 5 years. If it has not returned 10 years after treatment it is very unlikely to return.)

Source
http://www.macmillan.org.uk/Documents/AboutUs/Newsroom/LivingAfterCancerMedianCancerSurvivalTimes.pdf

How the chance of getting cancer has increased over time

Birth year	Lifetime risk : men	Lifetime risk : women
1930	39%	37%
1940	45%	43%
1950	50%	45%
1960	53%	47%

Source
"Trends in the lifetime risk of developing cancer in Great Britain: comparison of risk for those born from 1930 to 1960"
A S Ahmad, N Ormiston-Smith and P D Sasieni
British Journal of Cancer
3 February 2015
http://www.nature.com/bjc/journal/vaop/ncurrent/full/bjc201460
6a.html

Life expectancies

Year of birth	men	women
1930	59	63
1940	58	63
1950	66	71
1960	68	74
1970	69	75
1980	71	77
1990	73	79
2000	75	80

Source
Office for National Statistics

Costs

In 2010, the costs of cancer diagnosis and treatment across the UK NHS, private and voluntary sector were estimated by the report at £9.4 billion. This is equivalent to an average of £30,000 per person with cancer. Of this total expenditure, 85% is funded by the NHS, 9% is funded privately and the remaining 4% is funded by the voluntary sector.

Source
http://www.nhs.uk/news/2011/12December/Pages/cancer-treatment-cost-may-increase.aspx

NHS cancer spend

The largest (NHS) spending category in 2010/11 was mental health problems, accounting for 11% of the overall programme budget. Expenditure on circulatory problems was the second largest spend (7.2%), followed by cancers and tumours (5.4%). These three areas have represented the top three spending categories since 2004/05.

Source
http://www.nhshistory.net/parlymoney.pdf

Index

www.ingramcontent.com/pod-product-compliance
Lightning Source LLC
Chambersburg PA
CBHW070608290526
45790CB00002B/825